Live Better

alexander technique

13 DE

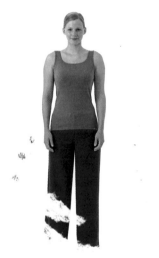

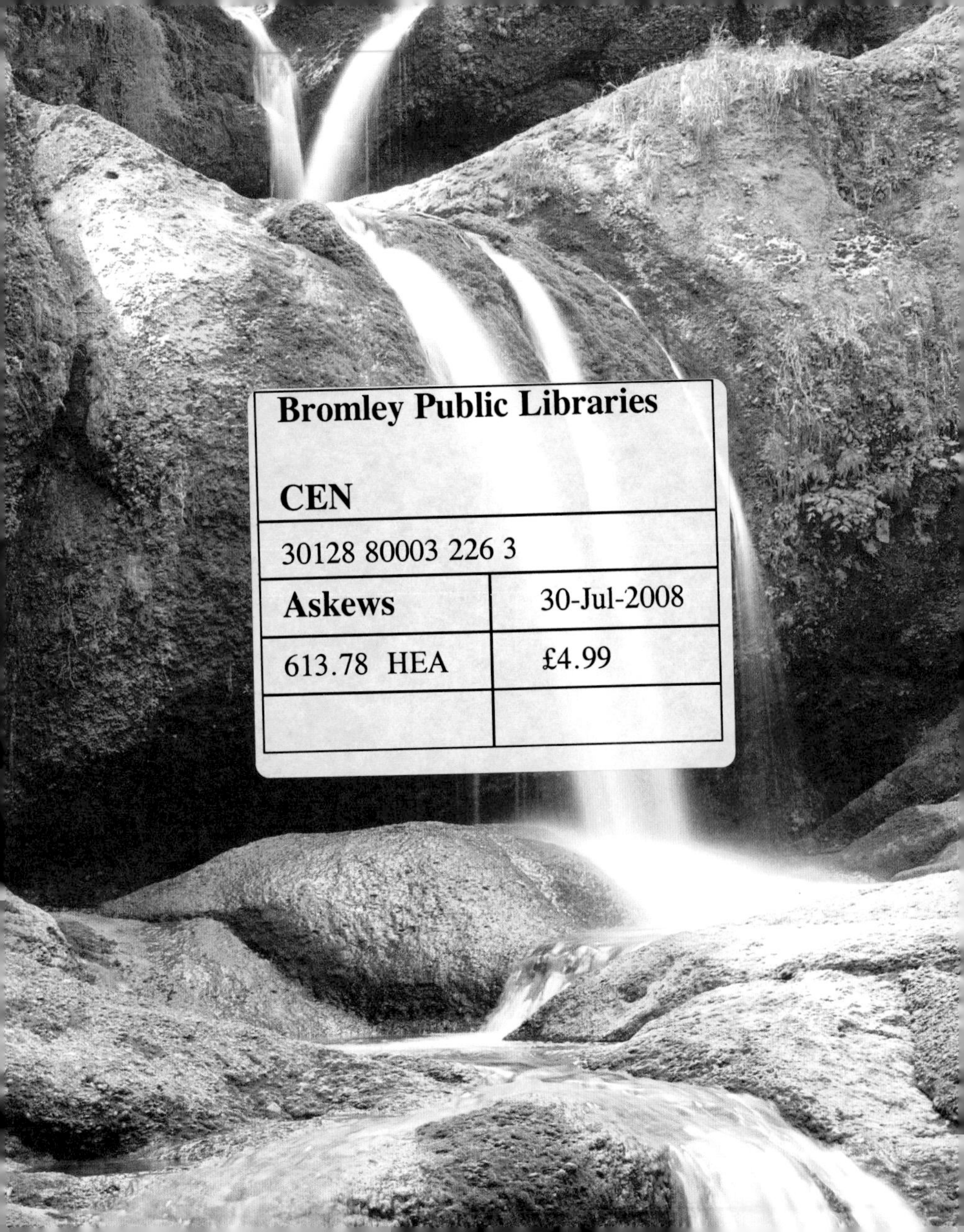

Live Better

alexander technique

skills and inspirations
for well-being

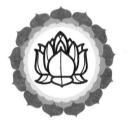

JOE SEARBY

DUNCAN BAIRD PUBLISHERS

LONDON

Live Better: Alexander Technique
Joe Searby

For Louise and Wilfred.

First published in the United Kingdom
and Ireland in 2007 by
Duncan Baird Publishers Ltd
Sixth Floor, Castle House
75–76 Wells Street
London W1T 3QH

Conceived, created and designed by
Duncan Baird Publishers Ltd

Managing Editor: Kelly Thompson
Editor: Susannah Marriott
Managing Designer: Daniel Sturges
Picture Research: Louise Glasson
Commissioned Photography: Matthew Ward

British Library Cataloguing-in-Publication Data:
A CIP record for this book is available from the
British Library.

10 9 8 7 6 5 4 3 2 1

ISBN: 978-1-84483-389-4

Typeset in Filosofia and Son Kern
Colour reproduction by Scanhouse, Malaysia
Printed and bound in Malaysia by Imago

Publisher's note
Before following any advice or practice suggested
in this book, it is recommended that you consult
your doctor as to its suitability, especially if
you suffer from any health problems or special
conditions. The publishers and author cannot
accept any responsibility for injuries or damage
incurred as a result of using any techniques
described or mentioned herein.

The abbreviations BCE and CE are used throughout
this book. BCE means Before the Common Era
(equivalent to BC); CE means of the Common Era
(equivalent to AD).

contents

Introduction 6

INTRODUCTION

The Alexander Technique is the most stimulating and life-changing discipline I have come across. It never ceases to inspire me, and its depth and potential grow for me every day. The Technique can be a challenging method to follow at first, but is never boring. It is subtle, but profound. Through this book I hope to inspire you to discover The Alexander Technique for yourself.

I first came across The Technique in 1983. In my work as a professional actor, I was seeking a discipline that would enhance my performance, yet offer something more profound than mere voice work or postural training. I began one-to-one Alexander lessons and soon realized that The Technique has effects that extend far beyond surface appearance (standing up straight) or physical cures (such as easing a bad back). I was lucky enough to start lessons at the age of 20, when I had no problems or pain (or so I thought). What surprised me the most were the psychological changes. The Technique fundamentally altered my outlook on life, changing me as a person: I believe it allowed me to become my true self. I have been teaching The Technique to others since 1995. For those willing to learn and apply its principles, The Alexander Technique is the only route to self-awareness and change I have encountered that gives you the skill to consciously direct your own energies.

This book introduces discoveries about the human condition made by F.M. Alexander more than 100 years ago, and sets out principles he developed while seeking an answer to his vocal problems (see pages 16–17). He refined his method over 60 years, laying down practices that remain cornerstones of the teaching.

Chapter One

origins and basics

The Alexander Technique is as unique and radical a method today as when Alexander first developed it in Australia in the early 1890s. You may be surprised to discover that such a cutting-edge bodywork system has been around for more than a century, and that the skills Alexander taught to others – which we still teach today – have not fundamentally altered in that time.

While working on himself to cure a voice problem that threatened his acting career, Alexander made key discoveries that can be applied universally to safe-guard human health. In essence, he established three findings: that mind and body are indivisible; that the way each of us manages ourselves as a whole person affects overall health; and that movement is governed by a centrally coordinated mechanism.

Don't be intimidated: The Alexander Technique is not a theory or hard-to-grasp philosophy, but a highly practical way to achieve personal development and physical change. This chapter explores Alexander's three principles in detail – each of them and other key terms are highlighted in sub-headings – looking at how he came to discover them, and why, as the pace of life accelerates, their implications are increasingly relevant to well-being. We look also at Alexander's life and offer a concise explanation of what The Technique is (and, just as importantly, what it is not).

WHAT IS THE
ALEXANDER TECHNIQUE?

The F. Matthias Alexander Technique, to use its full name, is a set of easy-to-learn practical skills. You apply them to how you use your whole "self" (mind and body) in every activity. As you move through life, you will want and need to learn new skills: to drive a car, play a musical instrument, speak another language, take up a sport or use a new tool. And daily demands require you to walk, lift, carry, sit, or use a computer. The common tool you require for these activities is yourself, and so the precursor to such actions – and all others – is learning how to "use" yourself. Until you have achieved this and can apply the skill to all activity, you are likely to get in the way of yourself, wasting energy, creating unnecessary wear, tear and strain on your body, and interfering with your ability to learn.

The skills of The Alexander Technique are methods of conscious thought and awareness: of thinking rather than doing. They do not require special equipment, and you don't have to isolate yourself from day-to-day life to practise them. You can apply them to every activity you might ever try, mental or physical. The skills are there for you to use in the act of living.

If we had to reduce The Technique to its essence, we could say that, at its simplest level, it teaches students how to release (and prevent) unnecessary, habitual muscular tension. Unwanted stiffening in the body's large muscles causes superfluous strain, wear and tear, and compression. It conflicts with balance, alignment and coordination, interfering with overall health and functioning, both physical and mental. The Alexander Technique teaches ways of applying the conscious mind that allow you to release this tension. Health, vitality and awareness then re-establish themselves naturally.

The Alexander Technique differs fundamentally from other mind–body disciplines, because it does not teach what to do and how to do it. Instead, it shows what not to do and how to prevent it, a simple process with far-reaching effects. The beauty lies in its practicality: you can start to use the skills from your very first lesson.

WHAT THE TECHNIQUE IS NOT

It may be easier to state what The Alexander Technique is not rather than what it is. First, it is not an alternative therapy or form of complementary medicine. There is no doubt that the benefits of The Technique can be hugely therapeutic, but it is not a therapy, as such, because it is not "done" to you. You are not a passive patient being treated, but an active student learning new skills.

The Alexander Technique is not an exercise regime, either, although applying its skills to activity, including exercise, is likely to make that activity more beneficial. Moreover, if you do *not* apply the skills, the benefits of exercise may be limited – or do more harm than good.

Neither is The Alexander Technique a bodywork method. It involves hands-on contact, but pupils are not massaged or manipulated. And despite relaxing both mind and body, The Alexander Technique is not a form of relaxation therapy either. In essence, The Technique is more than all these elements: it is a unique form of personal health education to transform your future.

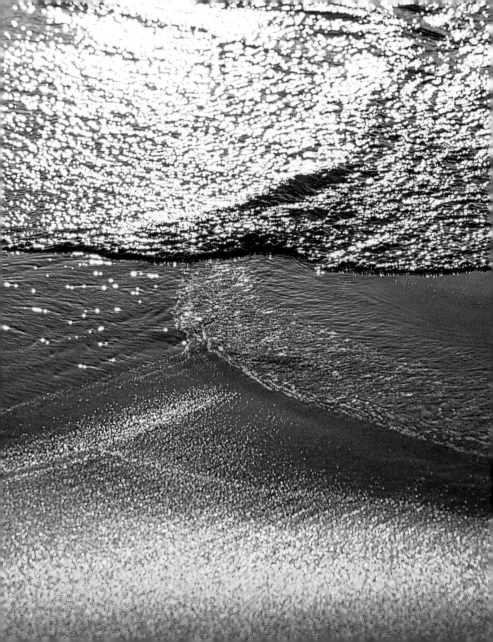

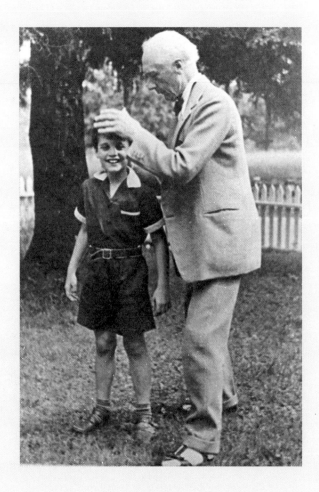

F.M. ALEXANDER:
A BRIEF BIOGRAPHY

The originator of The Technique – Frederick Matthias Alexander – was born in Tasmania, Australia, in 1869. He learned to ride when young, and a lifelong passion for horses and observing animals in their natural habitat informed his investigations into the human condition. So, too, did his refusal to accept the validity of anything he had not experienced personally. Aged 18, Alexander moved to mainland Australia, where he achieved his dream of becoming a professional actor. However, beset on stage by recurrent hoarseness, he began a journey of self-discovery that resulted in The Technique.

Seeking recognition for his method, Alexander moved to London in 1904 and soon found fame, thanks to the remarkable efficacy of his work. Here, he started writing four books that set out the nature of his system. They remain the basis of teaching today. During the two World Wars, Alexander took his work to the US. He taught until his death in London in 1955, aged 86.

ALEXANDER'S DISCOVERIES

Alexander discovered the principles of his method through personal experience. In his 20s, he found fame as an actor for the fine quality and dramatic dynamics of his voice. However, he suffered on stage from severe hoarseness and an audible sucking-in of breath, neither of which were conducive to a career in performance. Doctors found nothing wrong with his vocal mechanism, and no treatments were effective. So Alexander applied his talent for reasoning to the issue. He concluded that if nothing was wrong physically with his body's speech structures, the *way* he was using them must be causing the difficulties. He set out to pinpoint the problem.

Alexander assembled an arrangement of mirrors in which to observe himself from all angles, and began to rehearse in front of them, both speaking naturally and reciting lines. He saw that he was making all manner of effort unnecessary to the act of speaking, and that this became even more marked during recitation. Some of these mannerisms were legacies of attempts to carry out the instructions of his vocal or dramatic coaches. This insight led him toward his conclusion that specific training without reference to the whole person may not bring about improvement in a skill, and may even cause damage. In particular, Alexander saw that he contracted the muscles of his body strongly, notably in his neck and back. The resulting constriction throughout his system made speaking and reciting so difficult that it exerted tremendous strain on his voice, even when executing recommendations intended to make the recitation more effective. Worse, he found the stiffening habit so strong that he seemed unable to prevent it. Even when he felt he was preventing it, he could see that he wasn't.

By working on his personal problems patiently for several hours a day over many years, Alexander made discoveries fundamental not just to his own health and well-being, but to that of people the world over. He found that mind and body are indivisible, that the way we use this unified mind and body affects how well we function, and that the relationship between head, neck and back governs not just easy movement, but overall well-being.

THE WHOLE OF YOU
Psychophysical Unity

As you read these words are you using your mind or your body? Both, of course. Your fingers turn the pages, your eyes scan the words and your brain processes the data, allowing the mind to pass judgments. Reading is both physical and mental – what Alexander called a "psycho-physical" activity. When Alexander set out his principles in the early 20th century, the idea of mind–body unity was radical. Mind, body and spirit were usually regarded as three separate elements of the self. Although today we are used to connecting them, we still rank activity as physical or mental. What is playing tennis? How about chess? In one of his basic philosophies, Alexander states that every human activity is psychophysical – it involves the whole organism – and that treating mind and body as separate diminishes mental and physical health. When using the skills of The Alexander Technique, you consciously release undue physical effort, which brings about a return to mind–body unity.

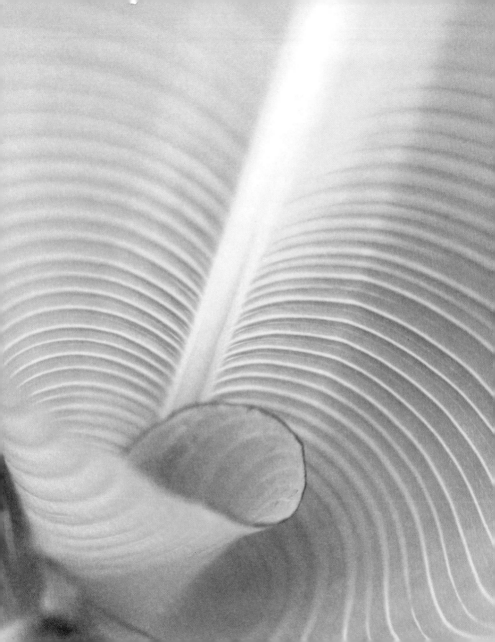

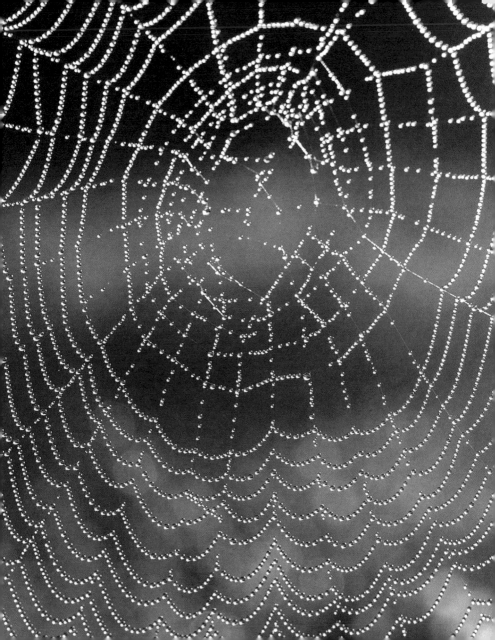

Unity in variety is the plan of the universe.

SWAMI VIVEKANANDA

(1863–1902)

Whoever holds in their mind the great image
of oneness, the world will come to them ...
in safety, oneness and peace.

LAO-TZU

(c.600–c.200BCE)

HEALTH AND WELL-BEING
Use and Function

Before using a complicated piece of equipment for the first time, you probably read the instruction manual. If you neglect this stage you may find that the equipment doesn't work as you expect when you press a key or run an incompatible program. The way you use equipment affects how well it functions. But do you know how to use the most important piece of equipment you possess: yourself? Human beings don't come with instructions: we trust that instinct will get us through. Another key Alexander principle teaches that if we don't "use" ourselves well, we don't function as well as we should: our back can hurt, breathing problems can develop, muscles stiffen or joints wear out; and we may become depressed, angry, or experience myriad other ailments.

Alexander was born prematurely and, from birth, he suffered periods of illness that forced him to rest for weeks at a time. In his 20s, as he began to address his vocal problems and devise ways of thinking that allowed him to undo the causes of this ailment, he saw remarkable results. Many other problems and ailments, which had hampered him since birth, also gradually disappeared. Alexander found that this was not peculiar to himself. When he taught his new-found skills to others, he saw marked improvements in their general health and well-being, not just in the symptoms that had motivated people to approach him. He thus confirmed that the way we "use" ourselves as a whole person affects how we function as an organism.

If you learn to use yourself well – by applying the skills of The Alexander Technique – you will function better and solve health problems in the process. Use yourself unconsciously, relying on habit, and you are likely to function poorly. For example, if you sit for long hours at the computer with a collapsed posture you may damage your back and put pressure on internal organs, hindering their function. Stiffening up is not a good option either: it creates unnecessary compression. You must learn to "use" yourself in a conscious way. Why not try the instruction of The Alexander Technique?

IT'S ALL IN YOUR HEAD
Primary Control

Take a moment to find something that weighs around 4.5–5kg (10–11lb). Sense how heavy it is. This is equal to the weight of your head, around eight percent of your total mass, sitting on top of your spine. Imagine pulling that weight down: it would start to squash your spine. If you also pulled it backward, it would drag you off balance. Yet Alexander saw that this is exactly what most of us get into the habit of doing: we contract our neck and back muscles, and pull the weight of the head back and down on the spine. He developed a way to prevent this habitual stiffening of muscles and to return to the natural alignment that can be seen in toddlers, as well as in adults who lead a more natural, often less westernized, lifestyle. In so doing, he found that a delicate, mobile relationship exists between the head, neck and back which works as a central coordinating mechanism for free, easy movement and optimal body functioning. Alexander named this principle the "primary control".

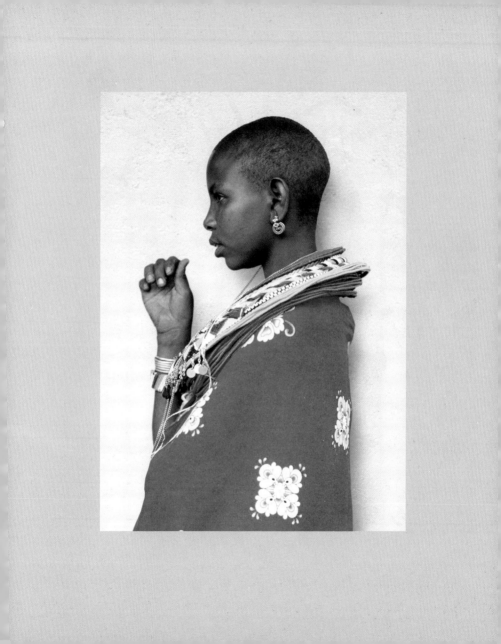

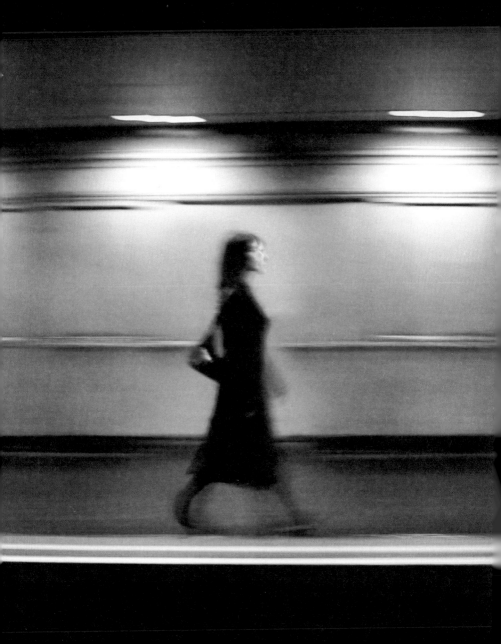

EXPERIENCING PRIMARY CONTROL

This practical exercise demonstrates how the "primary control" relationship between your head, neck and back works. Your spine has to lengthen through the centre of your body, like a firm spring. For this to take place, the weight of your head must move up, away from your body, to prevent it from compressing the spine. You can bring this about by consciously instructing, or "directing", the neck and back muscles to release unnecessary stiffening so they can lengthen and allow your back to open out.

Try projecting a series of "directions" (conscious orders) to your muscles by repeating, "I allow my neck to be free, which allows my head to move forward and up, which allows my spine to lengthen and my back to widen." Just project the orders; don't try to make anything happen. In a lesson, an Alexander teacher will encourage the muscles to release habitual tension with his or her hands as you give the internal orders, which is why The Technique works better, and results come more quickly, when you work one-to-one.

Happiness is when what you think,
what you say and what you do
are in harmony.

MAHATMA GANDHI

(1869–1948)

It's the whole, not the detail, that matters.

GERMAN PROVERB

Chapter Two

overcoming obstacles

The principles of The Alexander Technique provide solutions to challenges that are universal to human beings – challenges that manifest themselves in all of us to some degree and prevent us from fulfilling our potential. The originator of The Alexander Technique, F.M. Alexander, developed methods of thinking and acting that afford a way around key obstacles that can challenge us in many ways and affect everything from our careers to our health and our emotional lives.

The first obstacle Alexander recognized was that he was not always doing what he felt he was doing. This he attributed to "faulty sensory appreciation". Next, he found that his habitual way of acting – which he could see was causing damage – provided stronger stimulus than any new way of approaching an action. Finally, Alexander noticed that, because of his intense desire to reach goals, he was trying to attain results immediately, without regard to the best way of getting there. This concept he called "end-gaining". We all encounter similar barriers in daily life.

Alexander's answers to these obstacles are skills of conscious thinking that allow us to bypass or prevent problems. He referred to the skills as "direction" and "inhibition". This chapter discusses these and other key principles and skills of The Alexander Technique and shows how you can put them into action.

WHAT YOU FEEL
IS NOT WHAT YOU GET
Faulty Sensory Appreciation

We all have difficulty "feeling out" actions, such as the correct way to sit or stand. Indeed, a key principle of The Alexander Technique is that what we feel is not always what we get. Try this simple activity to test out the theory yourself. Stand next to a friend or face a mirror, taking your feet about hip-width apart. Close your eyes. Raise your arms out to the sides until they feel as if they are extending straight out from the shoulder, parallel to the ground. Take your time getting the action to feel right. Now open your eyes. Are your arms where you felt they were, or are they slightly out of line? Is one shoulder or arm higher than the other, or further forward? Adjust your arms, or have your friend adjust them, until they truly extend straight out from the shoulders, parallel to the ground. What does this feel like? Out of alignment or unbalanced? Simply wrong? Alexander named this inaccurate feeling "faulty sensory appreciation".

Alexander discovered faulty sensory appreciation by watching himself in a mirror. He noticed that he had strong muscular habits that caused him to stiffen and shorten, and saw that the habits were harming him. He identified one tendency as especially damaging: tensing his neck and compressing his head down onto his spine. Determined to do the opposite, Alexander worked for some time on extending his head upward. He sincerely felt as if he were getting it right, but when he looked in the mirror saw, to his astonishment, that he was still pulling his head down, the opposite action to the one he felt he was doing. When he began to observe and teach others, Alexander recognized that we all suffer from this faulty self-perception to some degree. We feel we are doing one action when we are actually doing another.

Understanding this concept sheds light on why we have difficulty "feeling out" actions: what we feel is right is actually wrong. It's like trying to navigate using a faulty compass. The hands-on guidance of an Alexander teacher helps us to find a conscious way of negotiating life without recourse to unreliable sensory perception.

GETTING WHAT YOU WANT
Direction

Do you desire a body that moves fluidly and functions with efficiency? To achieve this goal you have to let go of excess muscular tension, which causes compression and interferes with your natural expansion, alignment and balance. In his principle of "direction", Alexander teaches just how to do this.

To understand the principle, it helps to learn how important tension is to muscle function. For example, when you want to pick up an object, the biceps muscle in your upper arm receives a signal to contract. The muscle responds by increasing tension, shortening its length and raising your lower arm. Ask a muscle to act and there is an increase in tension. So any direct attempt to release a muscle and create natural expansion leads to tension and compression: the opposite effect to that intended. We require, instead, an indirect procedure. The indirect Alexander procedure to bring about muscular release and body alignment is known as "direction".

This skill entails sending conscious instructions to the body, then simply allowing unconscious systems to organize the action. At first, the orders will require the sensory input of a teacher's hands; otherwise, as Alexander found, we might think we are releasing tension or expanding when, in fact, we are doing the opposite.

Think of yourself as a ship. Your conscious mind is the captain on the bridge; your subconscious brain, nervous system and muscles are the crew. The captain gives the orders, but he can't run around performing all these actions himself: he lets the crew carry them out. In the same way, you can express your conscious wishes to your body and allow those wishes to be granted. If you want your neck muscles to release tension so that they stop pulling your head onto your spine, it's no good trying to *make* the release happen: this actually sends your muscles a signal to work harder. You should instead instruct your muscles to work less, make less effort, try less hard: to "not do". Then the muscles let go of any unwanted effort and lengthen, allowing your head to release in the desired direction.

EXPERIENCING DIRECTION

To feel the principle of "direction" in action, try this practical exercise with someone of a similar size. Sit on a regular-height chair (not a sofa) with your partner standing in front of you. Your partner takes you by the wrists and gently pulls you to your feet, being careful not to pull too hard or fast. Don't resist the pull. Ask your partner to make a mental note of the effort required. Now try again, but, before being pulled up, take a minute to think of yourself as incredibly heavy and stiff. Don't *do* this action, just really *think* it. Ask your partner how much more difficult it was to pull you up. Did your movement feel more uncomfortable?

Repeat the task, but this time thinking of yourself as incredibly light and mobile. Think of your head moving up and leading you onto your feet as your back becomes longer and wider. Ask your partner how much easier it was to pull you up. How much more pleasant was it for you? Swap roles so you both experience the difference. What created the difference? Simply, your thoughts.

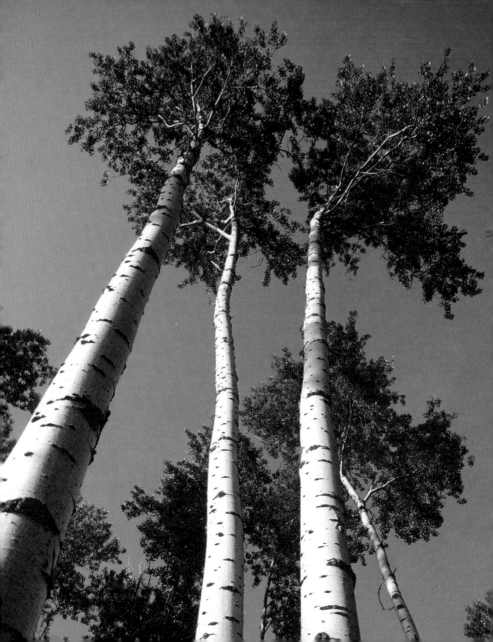

THE FORCE OF HABIT

How many times have you sat down? Or opened your mouth to speak? Or taken a step? Or bent down to pick something up? Countless times. But how often do you think about how you do those things? If you are like most people, then probably very rarely.

Because you have performed these actions (and so many others) so often, you have developed strong and unconscious habits that determine how you accomplish them. You're not aware of these habits, but they take over and often involve using too much muscular tension and effort. We all make more effort than necessary to tackle even very simple activities.

Right now take your attention to your hands. Are you holding this book lightly between your fingers or are you hanging on rigidly? What about your feet? Are they flat to the floor, or stiff and twisted around your chair? Are your toes gripping inside your shoes? Until you started to pay attention to these and other mannerisms, were you aware that you were doing them? Unfortunately not, and that's the problem with habits. We don't know we do them. What's worse, habitual tension distorts our awareness so that habits begin to feel right or normal and comfortable, even though they may be damaging us. Because our habitual "use" of ourselves is so strong and feels so right, it exerts a more powerful influence over us than any new way of acting. Our habits are what we know best and so to use ourselves without relying on habits is to step into the unknown.

Taking lessons in The Alexander Technique equips us with practical thinking skills that allow us to move away from the known and so to change muscular habits. In lessons, an Alexander teacher uses his or her hands to convey a sensory experience of moving through easy everyday activities without relying on habits of excess tension. At the same time the Alexander pupil is asked to give conscious orders, or directions, to reprogram muscle memory effectively. We learn through guided sensory experience to bypass comfortable but damaging habits, and this sets us up to step into the unknown with a new confidence and positivity.

EXPERIENCING YOUR HABITS

This practical exercise allows you to experience, perhaps for the first time, your unconscious habits. First face a mirror, standing with your arms hanging loosely by your sides. Fold your arms. Notice how your hands are placed; generally one hand rests on top of one arm and the other hand tucks under the opposite arm. Make a mental note of your preferred way of folding your arms. Let your arms hang down again. Now fold them the other way (with the opposite hand on top and the other hand tucked in). Make sure you really have reversed the arms. What does the action feel like? Awkward? Lopsided? Simply wrong?

Fold your arms again in your usual, habitual way. Note how easy the movement is and how right it feels. You don't have to think about it. Then reverse again, folding the non-habitual way. This requires conscious control and, even when you arrive in the pose, feels wrong, even though your arms may be anatomically identical. Unconscious habits exert a strong influence over all our actions.

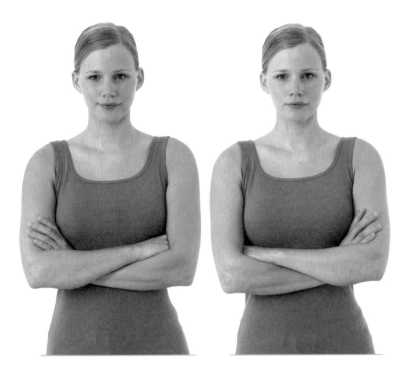

ACTING LIKE A CHILD
Stimulus and Response

What really excites or challenges you? The thought of swimming in open sea fills some people with dread, yet for others the same activity constitutes great fun. Those with a background in performance might find standing up in front of a hall of strangers exhilarating; for others this is the stuff of nightmares. That one person's stress is another person's stimulation proves that stimulus, or stress, itself is neutral. It is our reactions to stimuli that create difficulties.

Animals and small children react instinctively, or unconsciously, to stimuli. Seeing something attractive, they move toward it with tremendous ease and lack of effort. They don't have to think about how they move; unhindered movement is organized in reaction to the stimulus. They don't interfere with the natural "use" of themselves. However, as we grow older, we all develop patterns and habits in response to stimuli that interfere with that natural use. When responding to stimuli, we copy parents and siblings or adopt "cool" ways to use ourselves. Injury, emotional stress and muscular habits that stem from sitting at a desk, practising sport or other habitual actions also affect how we respond to stimuli. Habits and response patterns become deeply ingrained. Eventually when we move, speak or think in reaction to a stimulus, such as a demand, thought or need, we act on instinct and habit: a reaction that tends to involve excess effort. When this happens all day every day, it leads to problems. Alexander taught that instinctive behaviour no longer serves us well, as it causes us to have habitual reactions to stimuli. He saw that we need to be able to direct our reactions to prevent habitual responses, then consciously reason out an appropriate course of action.

This luxury of choice extends into emotional life, too. How often do you unthinkingly say yes to a request, when on reflection you would rather have said no? The Technique teaches how to create space between stimuli and your responses. You may still say yes, but having made a choice about how to react. Your reactions become, once again, as unhindered by habit as a child's.

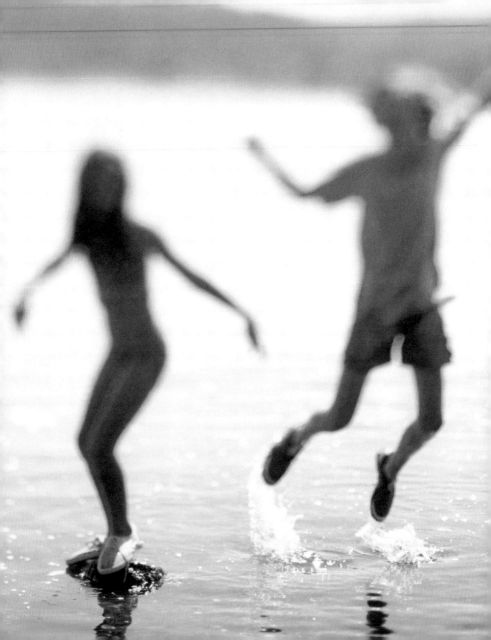

A truly great man never puts away
the simplicity of a child.

CHINESE PROVERB

Simplicity is the ultimate sophistication.

LEONARDO DA VINCI

(1452–1519)

FIGHT OR FLIGHT

Our most powerful and potentially damaging reaction
to a stimulus comes when we are faced with danger. In
such circumstances, animals, humans included, exhibit
a fight-or-flight response: the body produces a shot of
adrenaline (epinephrine), the heart and breathing rates
increase, and blood pressure rises as blood drains from
the skin to feed the large muscles. These reactions are
useful in the face of danger — a wild animal or speed-
ing car — because they prepare us to fight or take flight.
However, the fear reflex is not so useful when the stress
stimulus is ordinary and everyday: a deadline looming,
a traffic jam or a telephone ringing endlessly. Many
people exhibit an inappropriate fear response to daily
stresses, and so live in a state of unconscious anxiety.
It only takes a little more stress to tip the balance into
panic, agitation or rage. Apply the Alexander principle
of consciously reasoned reaction to a stimulus and you
maintain a level-headed distance from the stressor,
bringing about a more measured response.

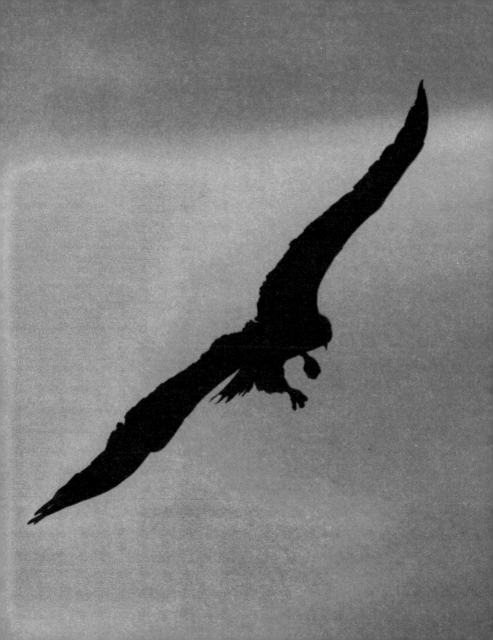

TENSION AND RELAXATION
The Middle Way

Although many of us believe that muscular tension is a bad thing, the body wouldn't get far without it. The problem with tension comes when we continue to hold it after it has finished its job. The Alexander Technique teaches that continuous, excessive tensing of the body's large muscles can distort the shape of the body, interfere with balance, and compress the spine and joints, leading to extra wear and tear and resistance to movement.

In order to understand how The Technique's skills work, it's useful to learn how two main types of muscle affect the way we move. Under the skin we wear a "suit" of muscles; let's call them movement muscles. They are quite large and strong: good for actions such as lifting, pushing, pulling, kicking and running. However, they don't have much stamina, working well over short bursts of activity, but tiring quickly. Deeper within, particularly around the joints of the skeleton and along the spine, is another set of muscles; let's call them support muscles.

They are not as strong as movement muscles but have almost limitless stamina and work continuously without tiring. Their function is to keep the body delicately poised upright in response to gravity's downward pull. The Technique knows them as "anti-gravity" muscles. It teaches that excessive habitual tension in movement muscles interferes with these support muscles and stops them from working. There are two consequences: either we fall or we use the body's movement muscles to hold us up. Naturally, we choose the second option, but the movement muscles tire easily, and so when we relax and release tension in large muscles, the support muscles don't work well and the body simply gives in to gravity.

People who don't follow The Technique tend to move between two unhealthy states: bracing big muscles to stay upright and "collapsing" into relaxing. Alexander teachers show how to release unwanted tension from the movement muscles and replace it with support from the anti-gravity muscles. Employing the skill of "direction" (see pages 34–35) releases stiff movement muscles while stimulating the anti-gravity muscles to wake up.

EXPERIENCING THE MIDDLE WAY

Calling on the support of the body's deep anti-gravity muscles offers a middle way between bracing muscles to stay upright and collapsing into "relaxation". You can experience "the middle way" with this practical exercise. Sit toward the front of a rigid chair and brace yourself into an upright position. Then try to stand and sense how the tension compresses you, making both movement and breathing difficult. Now sit again and let go of all the tension. Does your back slump backward? Does your upper body feel compressed? Is breathing easier? Sense how neither of these extreme postures is beneficial.

If you can do so comfortably, bend forward from the chair so your head hangs toward the ground. Let the neck relax. Slowly uncurl the spine to bring yourself upright. Ensure your head is the last part to return upright. As you arrive upright, continue to think of your head releasing toward the ceiling, your torso expanding outward from your spine. Sense your sitting bones on the chair. This is a taste of the "middle way" of anti-gravity support.

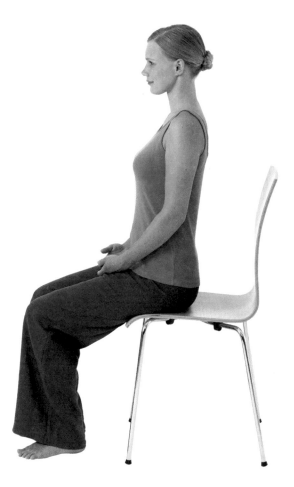

LESS IS MORE
Inhibition

In The Alexander Technique we work on preventing, or inhibiting, unnecessary tension caused by our habitual reactions to stimuli. It helps to be able to notice your own unique set of tensions. Try this practical exercise to start you thinking. Sit on an ordinary chair. Settle yourself, then consciously observe what happens if you slowly move to stand up. Do your legs stiffen and try to push your feet into the floor? Perhaps your arms swing forward or your shoulders tense up. Maybe you contract your neck and pull back your head.

The tensions you notice are your habitual reactions to the stimulus of standing up. Each of us has a personal collection of these reactions (as we do to all stimuli). But these habits of stiffening are unnecessary. They create potentially damaging compression throughout the body that makes movement more difficult. The Alexander Technique shows how to prevent such reactions and how to allow easier, more natural movement. We call this skill of prevention "inhibition". The term is not a negative one – try not to think of it as unconscious psychological repression – it means to prevent something unwanted from happening. This skill runs in parallel with that of "direction" (see pages 34–35), as follows:

First comes a wish, need or intention to do something, for example to sit, stand or speak. Usually we act on this intention habitually, or unconsciously. Deeply ingrained pathways from the subconscious brain to the muscles are activated, triggering unwanted stiffenings. The Alexander Technique teaches us to think in a way that "inhibits" the activation of these pathways, and at the same time shows how to project conscious directions for overall release, especially of the head, neck and back. Then we allow natural movement to happen.

The key to inhibition is awareness – mindfulness of habits as you perform them – for until we become aware of something, we can't do much about it. Being consciously aware brings the possibility of change. This means that The Technique becomes a practical tool for achieving more by consciously doing less.

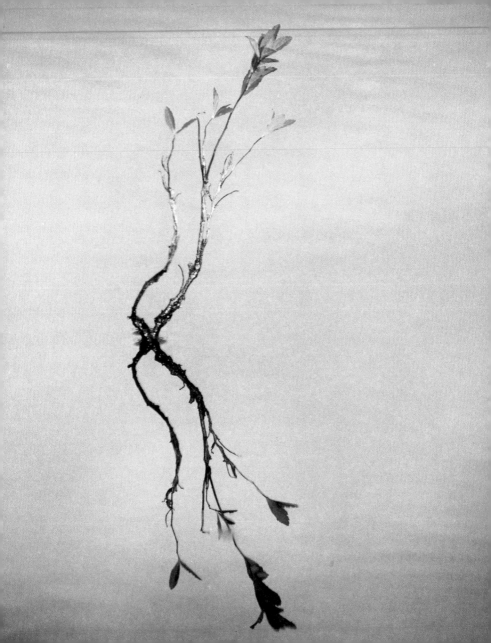

If you can stop doing the wrong thing,
the right thing does itself.

F.M. ALEXANDER

(1869–1955)

The first point of wisdom is to discern what is false;
the second to know what is true.

LACTANTIUS

(c.240–c.320ᴄᴇ)

GOING FOR IT
End-gaining

With slogans like "Go for it" and "Just do it", consumer culture gears us up for hasty action and reaction, urging us to rush toward and achieve goals at any cost, without paying attention to how we get there. More than 100 years ago, Alexander identified this universal tendency; today's increased pace of life has only intensified the problem. Alexander called the habit "end-gaining", and the skills of The Alexander Technique teach ways to inhibit this unthinking desire to get what we want right away. In so doing, we discover that the quality of the end result is connected to the quality of the process.

Alexander teachers work with you as you perform habitual actions, such as sitting, standing and lifting, to help you spot small-scale end-gaining. This equips you to recognize and prevent longer term end-gaining, which can negatively affect health and well-being. In this way The Technique enables you to live fully in the present, rather than trying to end-gain the future.

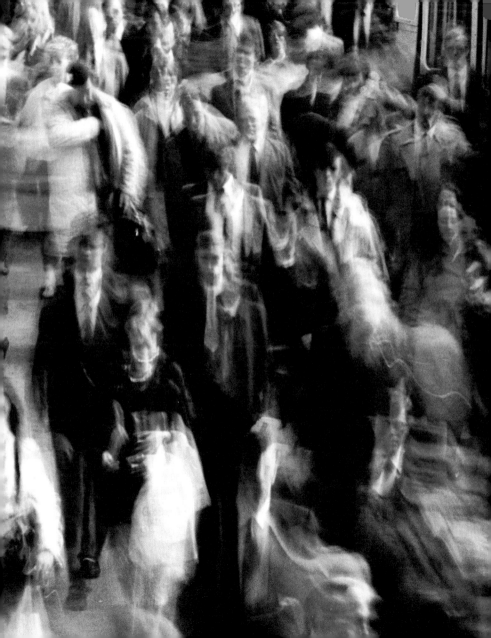

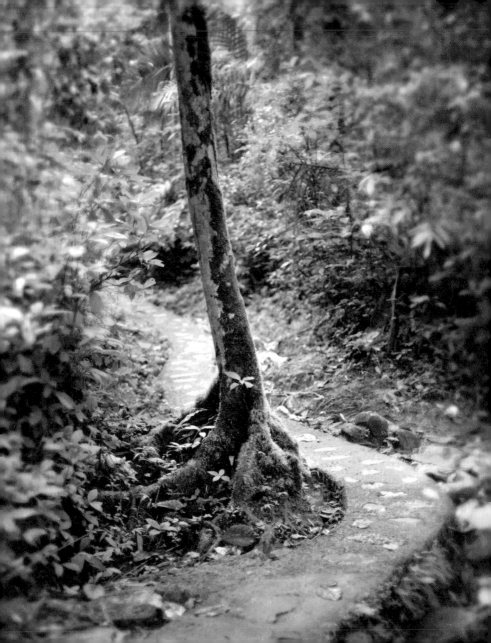

THE JOURNEY, NOT THE DESTINATION

The practice of mindfulness is a core tenet of many philosophies of living. It involves being aware of thoughts and actions in the present, rather than falling into the habitual trap of dwelling on the past or dreaming of what might be. Within these disciplines you might be required to remove yourself from daily life to develop the skill of mindfulness, perhaps through meditation.

Alexander developed an eminently practical means of attending to the present, applied not in an esoteric practice, but in every action. When you bring conscious attention to your "use" of yourself in activity, even the simplest undertakings become opportunities to practise mindfulness. By employing the skills of "direction" (see pages 34–35) and "inhibition" (see pages 52–53), you move toward being in the now and open up your field of awareness, as you free the body from damaging habitual tension. To live in the moment all you need to do is allow the skills of The Technique to direct your attention to the process of activity, rather than the end you wish to gain.

Have patience with all things,
but chiefly have patience with yourself.
Do not lose courage in considering
your own imperfections, but instantly
set about remedying them –
every day begin the task anew.

ST FRANCIS DE SALES

(1567–1622)

The journey is the reward.

CHINESE PROVERB

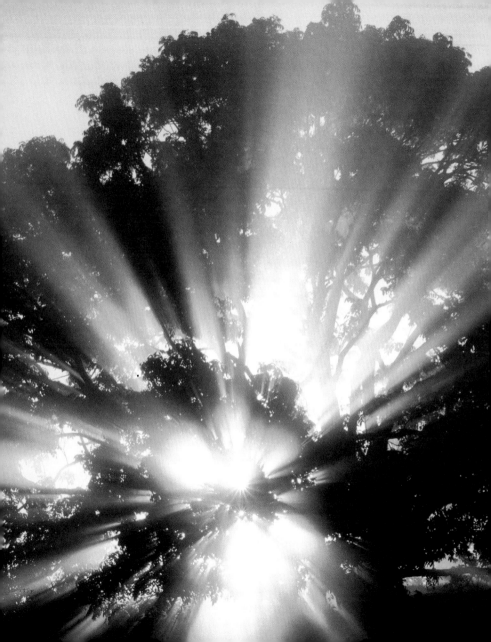

Chapter Three

why turn to The Alexander Technique?

Learning and applying the skills of The Alexander Technique can enhance every aspect of your life. If this claim sounds ambitious, consider what The Technique teaches. You learn how to consciously direct the ways in which you use every part of yourself – mind and body – and you coax those elements to work together as a whole. Any aspect of yourself can therefore be coached to function more effectively, from how you move to the ways in which you think. Of course, people don't often turn to The Technique in order to change their entire life. Many seek out its skills for specific reasons, often in response to a symptom, such as a bad back, although Alexander teachers are, on the whole, not qualified to treat specific medical conditions. Other people approach a teacher to enhance skills in a particular activity, from sport to playing music. Some begin lessons for stress-relief, to build energy or to prevent future problems. Reasons for coming to The Technique are as varied as each of our personalities. This chapter assesses some of the most common motivations and demonstrates how The Alexander Technique can help in diverse circumstances.

REDUCING AND PREVENTING PAIN

Many Alexander teachers report that pain is pupils' primary motivation for learning The Technique. Pain is a great motivator; indeed, many people don't become aware of a health problem until something starts to hurt. Pain is often the body's way of shouting for attention – and is commonly a local manifestation, or symptom, of a more generalized problem. Many of us respond to pain by ignoring it, or resting, then returning to the activity that caused it. This is not the Alexander approach.

The Alexander Technique has a strong track record in treating pain that results from long-term muscular tension, notably of the neck and back. This encompasses a range of painful joint and skeletal disorders, but lower back pain is a common example. When back pain results from unnecessary curvature and compression of the lumbar (lower) spine, the cause may be habitual over-contraction of the body's large muscles. Rest can bring a temporary relief of pain, but cannot undo the habitual stiffening that is its cause. Alexander skills show you how to undo this compression and allow a natural expansion throughout your body. Learning to regain natural poise in this way brings relief from pain. More importantly, it wipes out the cause of the problem. Alexander's focus on the causes of pain, not simply the symptoms, distinguishes his work from other therapeutic disciplines, which tend to take a more symptomatic approach to health and well-being.

If you have suffered chronic pain for many years, see a doctor before approaching an Alexander teacher and be aware that pain is unlikely to disappear overnight, although painful habits often change quickly with The Technique and never take as long to undo as they did to create. One of the first lessons of The Technique shows ways to release unwanted muscular tension and realign the head, neck and back. You can gain relief from a host of painful symptoms in the process.

Prevention is better than cure. If you study The Technique from an early age, you learn to use yourself well before pain starts, thus effortlessly avoiding what many consider to be an inevitable part of life.

IMPROVING POISE AND POSTURE

Pupils beginning The Alexander Technique often hope to improve their posture. But what is "good" posture? Common instructions command us to stand up straight, pull back the shoulders and draw in the stomach. The concept of having to hold the body in "correct" poses seems universal. But an Alexander teacher shows how holding the body in a fixed position requires excess muscular effort, which puts unnecessary compression and strain on your body's system.

To experience the tension inherent in what many may regard as good posture, stand up straight and fix yourself into a classic parade-ground stance. Or think of yourself as a debutante, standing with a pile of books on your head, trying not to let them fall. Now take a walk. Does holding yourself in either of these "good" postures help or hinder you? Watch whether you have to let go of most of the tension before you can move. What happens to your breathing? The body is designed to move: fixed poses and motion are incompatible. To see the concept in action, watch an animal or child moving. They don't hold themselves. They maintain natural poise, not a fixed pose. Poise is about finding freedom and balance, coordination, and a readiness to move. It is not about stiffening the back in order to stay upright. The Technique teaches practical ways to regain a natural, upright poise and maintain the free balance, coordination and mobility of your whole self as you move. The principles teach you how to consciously release any stiffening that interferes with that natural use. One of the benefits is that other people will notice your improved posture. But what you really gain – or regain – is natural poise: the free poise you had as a small child before excess habitual tension got in the way.

We understand intuitively that our state of mind is reflected in our physical stance, and vice versa: think of how many descriptive phrases, such as "feeling down" or "having the weight of the world on our shoulders" make the link. Learning to free tension from the body and achieve natural poise also makes possible a more easy and balanced emotional life.

EXPERIENCING POISE

This exercise gives a flavour of how an Alexander teacher works with a pupil to re-establish natural poise, although when you work with a teacher you also gain non-verbal, hands-on input. Stand with your feet about hip-width apart, arms hanging loosely by your sides. Sense the ground beneath your feet. Don't think of the ground as something that stops you falling to the centre of the earth, but as an active force that lifts you. Bring your attention to the top of your head and think of allowing it gently to rise away from the soles of your feet. Consciously stretch yourself, creating space in the joints of the body: your ankles, knees, hips and the top of your spine.

Having regained some natural expansion, feel free to carry it into movement. Why not go for a walk? Let your eyes find an attractive object and lead you toward it. As you move, allow expansion out from the centre of your body. You should sense increased lightness, a result of your conscious thought. The hands-on help of a teacher enhances and speeds such releases.

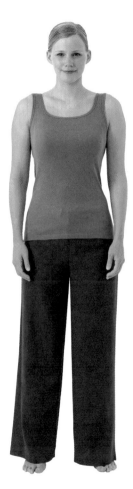

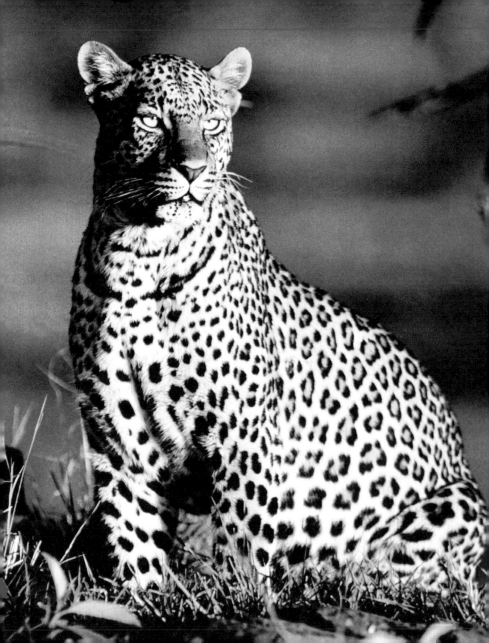

Let us be poised, and wise, and our own, today.

RALPH WALDO EMERSON

(1803–82)

Grace has been defined as the outward expression
of the inward harmony of the soul.

WILLIAM HAZLITT

(1778–1830)

RELEASING TENSION

Many of us seek release from physical tension and stress via relaxation techniques. Although approaches such as meditation and massage may ease anxiety and unknot stiffness, they cannot change the stiffening habits of muscles. The skill of releasing muscular tension lies at the heart of The Alexander Technique. Moreover, when you work with an Alexander teacher, you learn that there is no distinction between physical tension and mental stress. Because there is no separation, releasing need-less habitual muscular effort brings about a reduction in mental – and even spiritual – distress.

Applying the principles of The Technique to undo muscular habits and their outcome (mental agitation) begins a virtuous circle. Having a quiet mind makes you less likely to stiffen in response to stress, and so you ease habitual mental responses of tension and anxiety and may stop dwelling on issues that worry you and cause strain. Best of all, you employ these skills in the act of living rather than in the isolation of a relaxation class.

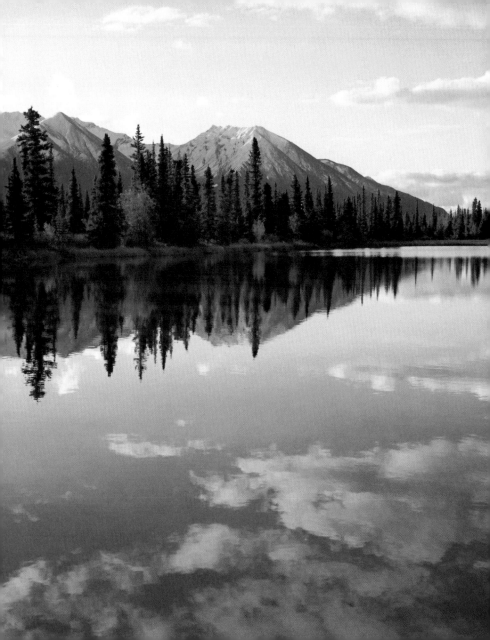

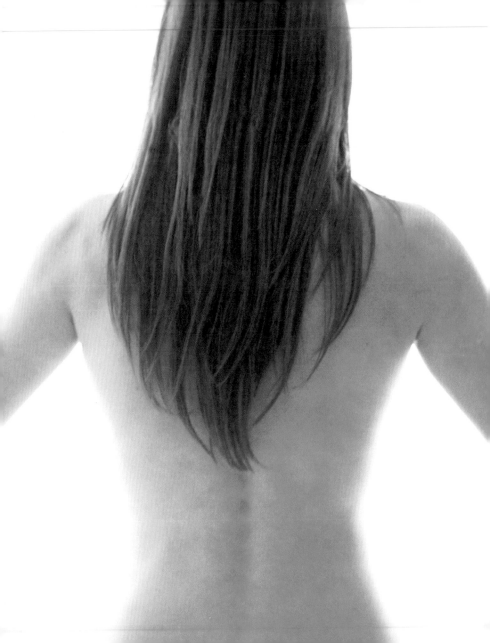

STRENGTHENING THE BACK

Back pain is a widespread motivator and many people turn to an Alexander teacher because of this symptom. But Alexander teachers look at the whole person rather than at symptoms – they are interested in "coherence" between the various parts of a pupil. Back-pain sufferers may be pleased to learn that the key coordinating factor in this coherence is the strength of the back.

What makes a strong back? Stiff, overdeveloped muscles? No, these simply cause contraction. A super-bendy spine? No, this fails to support adequately. Think of the spine neither as stiff and rigid nor floppy and bendy, but as a firm, lengthening spring. The Technique shows how to create an even-toned, elastic musculature to support the spine and allow it to function effectively. By applying conscious thought, you permit back muscles to release excess tension so they open out, rebalance in tone and allow the spring of your spine to extend through the centre of your body. Then you achieve strength, poise and endurance, as well as freedom from back pain.

GETTING THE MOST FROM EXERCISE

Exercise is beneficial in many ways: the fitness benefits of boosted circulation and breathing are accompanied by the psychological advantages of taking part in a pastime that you enjoy, and feeling good about yourself. Exercise is most effective when you engage your mind as well as your body in the activity. Then you master skills faster, achieve better results, and injuries become less likely. Applying the principles of The Alexander Technique makes sure you engage your mind. Alexander teachers work with you on ways to use your mind to undo habits of tension in the body, so permitting your whole self to operate as freely as possible during activity.

The Alexander Technique is especially useful for those of us with sedentary lives who separate exercise from work and other day-to-day tasks, and who seek to make amends by joining a gym or attending fitness classes. Imagine you have the habit of stiffening your neck and pulling the weight of your head back and down onto your spine, interfering with your body's overall coordination (as most of us do, most of the time). Does this habit disappear when you exercise? Unfortunately not. Indeed, the more demanding an activity, the more exaggerated habits tend to become. Now picture joining a gym to get fit, perhaps because your weight is on the increase and you have lower back pain. You go to the gym and start using its array of machines, taking toning classes and lifting weights. But your unconscious habit of stiffening and contracting muscles when performing even very simple actions is still with you. In fact, it gets worse. Every time you use a weights machine or take a class, you increase effort and compression throughout your system. Your muscles develop impressively, but is the exercise doing you good or harm in the end?

The same question can be asked about any sport, from golf to tennis, soccer to cycling, where long-held patterns of unnecessary tension can hinder skills and performance and may lead to damage. Remember there is nothing wrong with exercise itself: just be certain you are not exercising your bad habits. When you work with The Technique you can be sure that you are not.

ENHANCING THE ATHLETE

Many high-achieving sportspeople naturally use their key piece of sporting equipment – themselves – well. This "use" is often instinctive, or unconscious; they don't know how it works, it just does. Other athletes succeed despite using themselves poorly, getting by on sheer willpower and determination (and often paying a price in the form of injury). Both types of sportsperson, however, would benefit from learning The Technique.

When sudden and unexplained loss of technique hits naturally gifted athletes, it can be very difficult for them to regain form if they are unaware of the source of their innate skills. Alexander methods, however, can be applied consciously, so athletes can return to them again and again to maintain and improve performance, as well as to regain technique should they lose it.

Athletes who succeed through sheer force of will and effort often find that The Technique helps to reduce the work they have to put in to achieve the same or better results, and, on the way, helps to avoid injury.

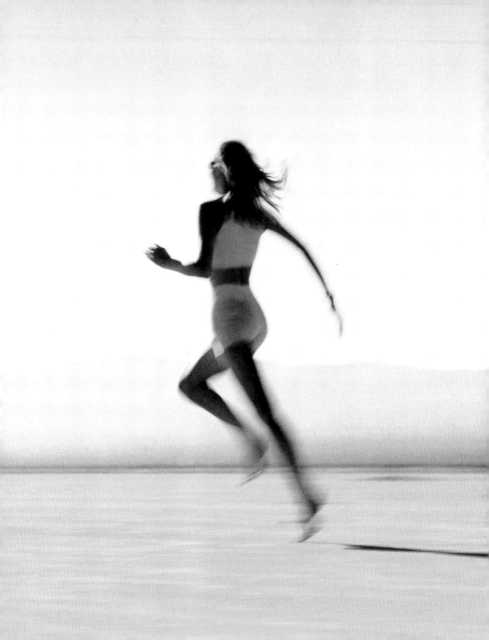

BOOSTING PERFORMANCE

The Alexander Technique was born out of one man's need to remedy a performance-related problem that threatened his stage career. Since its very inception, The Technique has therefore enjoyed strong links with the performing arts. Today, it is taught in music colleges and drama schools around the world, and performers of all types benefit from applying its principles.

Acting

You can use The Technique if you are an actor, just as its originator did, to improve the quality of your voice and the way in which you use it. But acting is more than being able to speak well. Much of the impact an actor makes on an audience, whether on stage or through the camera, derives from their "presence". This somewhat mystical quality might be described as an ability to be completely self-assured and "in the moment", something from which all performers benefit. The Alexander skill of consciously directing energy maximizes stage presence.

Dancing

In dance the whole person becomes your instrument of expression. When you apply the skills of The Alexander Technique to this instrument you not only reduce the risk of injury, but free the body from unwanted tension. This allows a more direct translation of your conscious intent into physical result.

Presenting for business

Giving a business presentation to a group of colleagues or clients can be as nerve-racking for some people as walking onto a stage. Getting a point across while being entertaining is stressful if you don't have a background in performance. Stress can cause you to stiffen up, stop breathing, suffer a dry throat and even lose your nerve. It also negatively affects your posture. Confidence and good posture go hand in hand, and positive body language plays a huge role in communication. Alexander skills present practical ways to use conscious, positive thinking to improve your physical and mental attitude, and so enhance your delivery and overall performance.

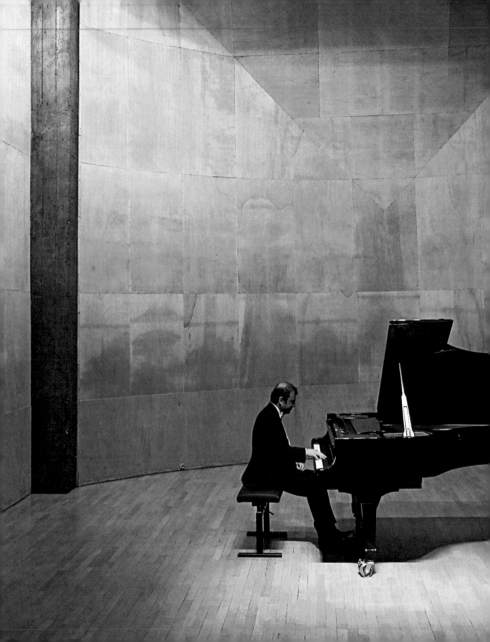

Giving a speech

How many times have you seen someone give a reading and strained to hear as they mumbled into the lectern or raced through from sheer terror? An Alexander teacher guides you through simple ways to slow down, become audible and make the most of your chance to perform.

Performing music

One of the greatest obstacles to continuing success in the performing arts is unnecessary effort. For instrument players this can be especially damaging, even leading to career-threatening tension and pain. Alexander skills help you to cope better with the great physical and mental demands of playing an instrument, and while reducing the risk of injury, also improve your quality of sound.

Singing

Quality of voice is paramount for singers because your "instrument" directly translates your intention into sound. Alexander skills make available the full breath and vocal freedom that comes when blockages are released.

FREEING THE BREATH

While shallow breathing is unlikely to be your reason for seeking an Alexander teacher, our breathing is, in fact, the first of the body's natural processes to be affected when we carry tension. The negative consequences for your health – physical and mental – might, therefore, lead you to a teacher. The Alexander Technique is very effective at freeing parts of the breathing apparatus that may have become restricted by tension to allow a deeper and more natural flow of air in and out of the body.

To witness the way tension can disrupt natural breathing patterns, try a simple exercise. Focus as hard as you can on this word: "breathe". Watch your breath. Does it slow or even stop? Perhaps it feels a little more constricted than before? If so, this shows that excessive effort creates tension, which obstructs easy breathing. The Alexander Technique teaches us how to diffuse such unnecessary effort and stop interfering with the breath. It allows us not to "do" breathing, and permits unconscious mechanisms to work once again and organize it for us.

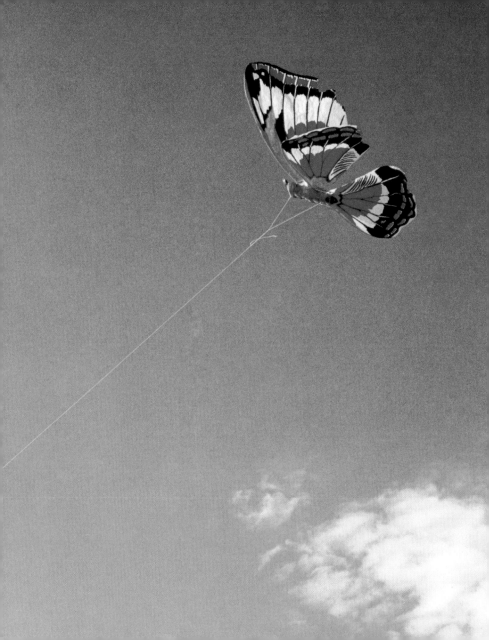

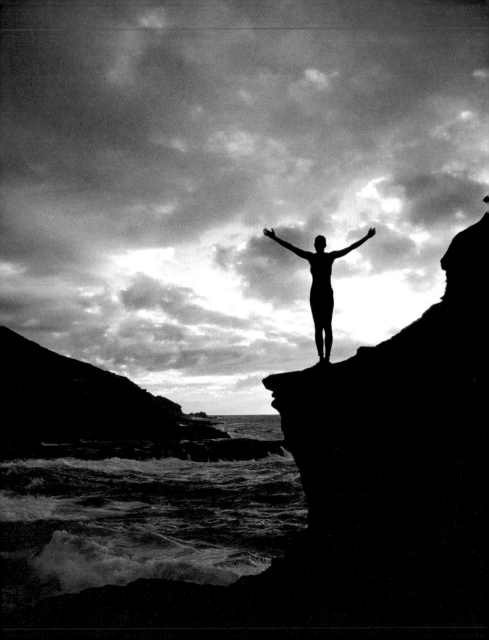

The miracle is not to fly in the air, or to walk on the
water, but to walk on the earth.

CHINESE PROVERB

Men go abroad to wonder at the heights of mountains,
at the huge waves of the sea, at the long courses of the
rivers, at the vast compass of the ocean, at the circular
motions of the stars, and they pass by themselves
without wondering.

ST AUGUSTINE

(354–430CE)

BUILDING ENERGY

The demands of modern living mean we often wish we had extra energy to get us through the day. Alexander skills help us to reclaim energy expended in contracting muscles unnecessarily. Specifically, skills of "direction" (see pages 34–35) and "inhibition" (see pages 52–53) teach us how to release and prevent habitual effort, freeing a good deal of energy to put to better use. Pain caused by stiffening is draining, too; applying The Technique brings about pain reduction, thus boosting energy.

It may help to think of direction as the ability to channel energy consciously to where it is needed in the way it is needed. Disciplines such as yoga or tai chi call this life-force energy *prana* or *chi*. Whichever name you use, with Alexander skills you liberate this energy to prevent blocks, or organize it to stop it dispersing.

Resistance to illness – "vital capacity" – depends on how well your digestion, circulation and breathing work. Improving your use of yourself enhances the efficiency of these functions to raise energy levels and immunity.

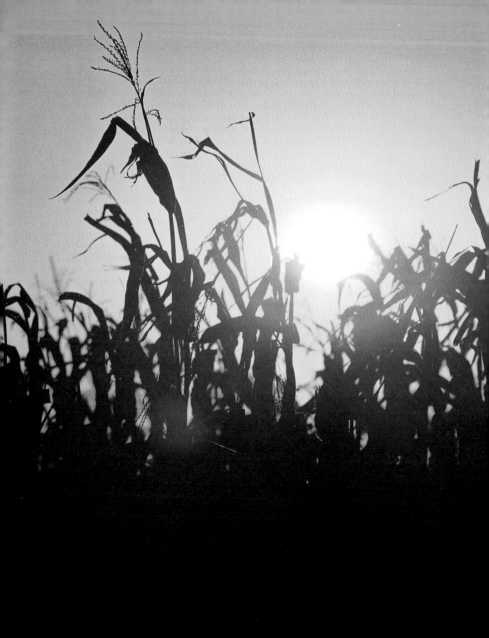

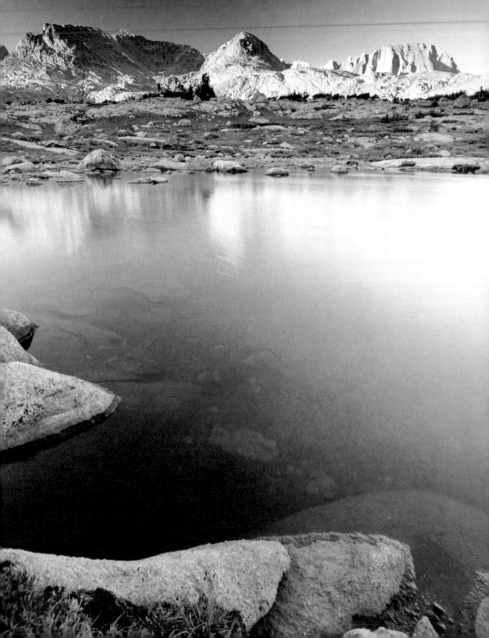

Everything is extraordinarily clear. I see the whole
landscape before me. I see my hands, my feet, my toes,
and I smell the rich river mud. I feel a great sense
of strangeness and wonder at being alive.

THE BUDDHA

(c.4TH CENTURY BCE)

Chapter Four

visiting a teacher

The Alexander Technique comprises a total sensory experience. Words simply cannot convey how it feels to experience the new you that emerges when you stop relying on habitual ways of moving and thinking and return instead to "natural" ways of being. Imagine describing a sensory experience, perhaps the sound of a lamb bleating or the colour of a flower, to someone who has never heard a lamb or seen the colour. Would any number of words be adequate to describe that sensation? How much more effective it would be to let the person hear the sound or see the flower. The experience would then be complete and undeniable, understood in a way impossible through description alone. It would be a "psychophysical" – total sensory – event. Similarly, reading about The Technique can only ever be a description. Having a lesson with an Alexander teacher is like hearing the lamb or seeing the colour for yourself. You need the hands-on input of an Alexander teacher to lead you out of your known world and into the unknown in order to sense a new you, freed from past experience and recurring habits.

This chapter explores what to expect from lessons in The Technique and what to look for in a teacher. It examines the specialized way teachers use their hands, and shows how applying the skills can support daily activities, such as sitting, standing and walking.

DO I REALLY NEED A TEACHER?

You may wonder why this book doesn't present you with a programme to follow. The reason is that you are an individual, different from any other person walking this planet. And, as an individual, you have assembled a personal collection of habits and tension patterns as you have moved through life. They may be similar in some ways to those of other people, but at the core you are who you are. So how could we write a single course in The Technique that works not only on your habits, but on those of every other reader, too?

It is possible to study practical skills – such as golf or driving – from a book or online. But if you do so, you may not be surprised when you acquire unhelpful and unnecessary habits. These come about because faulty sensory appreciation (see pages 32–33) prevents us from adequately correcting ourselves, and force of habit imprints unproductive ways of doing things on body and mind. Similarly, learning The Technique without the aid of a teacher would at best be slow and problematic, and at worst doomed to failure. Alexander writes in the introduction to *The Use of the Self*, "It took me years to reach a point that can be reached in a few weeks with the aid of any experienced teacher." A teacher works on your individual pattern of habits and muscular tension, and offers hands-on input: the only way to real change.

What about group learning? Introductory group workshops offer a good induction into the ideas of The Technique, and enable you to make an informed choice about whether to opt for one-to-one lessons. However, in a group environment you may not get much hands-on contact, making ongoing group work a false economy. Alexander taught his Technique for 60 years, but only ever one-to-one. It wasn't that the originator found groups difficult – he was an actor; he just understood the nature of human problems and saw that change comes only when you work on an individual basis. Alexander was eager that as many people as possible should reap the benefits of "the work". If he had thought it possible to pass on benefits in large groups or by correspondence courses, I'm sure he would have done so.

FINDING A TEACHER

When choosing an Alexander teacher, first look for someone who has completed an approved training, even if he or she has chosen not to join a professional body. STAT (The Society of Teachers of the Alexander Technique) is the largest representative body for Alexander teachers. Founded in 1958, STAT is based in the UK, but societies around the world are affiliated to it. This body maintains and enforces codes of professional conduct, and ensures members are fully insured.

It's best to find a teacher local to home or work. To source details of teachers working in your area, contact the STAT-affiliated organizations on page 128. Book introductory lessons with two or three teachers. When learning The Technique, it is important to establish good communication with a teacher. If one teacher doesn't work, try another. You wouldn't blame a keyboard if you didn't get on with a piano teacher, so it's best not to dismiss The Alexander Technique if you fail to establish a rapport with one or more teachers.

Training to become an Alexander teacher is a great commitment, and pupils are often surprised to discover just how long it takes. Alexander started his first teacher training course in London in 1931. Several of the first teachers to qualify with Alexander in the 1930s set up courses. In turn, people they trained established schools, preserving a direct line of tradition from the originator right across the world. Today, there are teacher training courses from Argentina to Australia and from Belgium to Brazil. The model Alexander used is still followed by most: a minimum of 1,600 hours' tuition over three years. The commitment translates to around three hours' study a day, five days a week for 36 weeks a year over three years. Because of the amount of time and money required of a teacher in training, most courses are small in scale. Class size is dictated also by the highly practical nature of the training: nearly all the work is "hands-on", requiring a ratio of at least one teacher to five students. Qualification is by continuous assessment. This should reassure you about the commitment your teacher has to the discipline and to you, the pupil.

THE TEACHER'S HANDS

You are in safe hands with Alexander teachers. They use their hands to gather information about your body's structure, alignment and ways of working, assessing where there is undue tension or not enough tone. In this sense a teacher's hands work as receivers. At the same time they act as transmitters, encouraging change and aiding the release of excess muscular tension to bring about natural realignment. This touch is not a form of manipulation; more a manual guiding. So while the teacher's hands listen, they also speak, imparting knowledge to the body at a non-verbal level. Most of the information a pupil receives in a lesson is unspoken. Such direct and non-verbal communication of sensory experience sets The Technique apart from bodywork disciplines that promise postural improvement. It also explains why a teacher needs "good" hands: energized yet soft, open and able to impart positive experience. The only equipment Alexander teachers require is their hands. So they can teach you anywhere, any time.

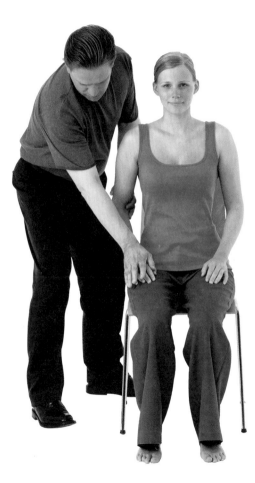

WHAT TO EXPECT FROM A LESSON

When you arrive for your first lesson in The Alexander Technique, don't expect to find a practitioner in a white coat working in a clinical setting. Although teachers tend to have a broad knowledge of medical conditions, they are not doctors. Nor should you anticipate a classroom situation. Although they may call themselves teachers and refer to you as a student, similarities between The Technique and other forms of formalized education end there. Try to leave preconceptions about healthcare and learning at the door, and enter with an open mind.

Most Alexander teachers offer lessons lasting either 30 or 40 minutes, according to personal preference. This tends to be the optimum learning time. Longer times can be counterproductive, overloading a pupil with verbal and sensory information. Wear ordinary, comfortable clothing, although trousers may be more suitable than a skirt. You will not need to remove items other than shoes. Nor will you be manipulated in any invasive way. Although powerful in effect, the hands-on contact from an Alexander teacher is gentle and subtle. Teachers tend to combine hands-on contact with a variety of strategies to bring you to awareness of your habits. These will vary according to the teacher, his or her experience and your interests, but some of the core activities that everyone who comes to learn The Technique will experience are explored on pages 102–119.

Because individual needs vary, it is unwise to try to specify exactly how many lessons you might require and how often, but broadly, 25 to 30 lessons over about six months should equip you with sufficient grounding in The Technique to take away the principles and apply them yourself. Many people notice significant change within a few lessons. I usually suggest that pupils attend lessons twice a week for a few weeks and once a week thereafter. The best advice is to try a lesson and then discuss your personal needs with the teacher.

Please note that Alexander teachers have no medical qualifications as such (unless they trained in medicine) and therefore cannot make diagnoses. If you have health concerns, consult your doctor as well as a teacher.

WHAT YOU MIGHT DO IN A LESSON

In every Alexander teacher's workspace you will find two objects: a table and a chair. The table is designed for bodywork, but the chair is often ordinary. "Chair work" and "table work" are core activities in most Alexander lessons. Lying on a table, or sometimes on the floor, is looked at in more detail on pages 116–119. In chair work the teacher asks you to sit on a chair and rise from it. As you do so, he or she helps you to become aware of strong habits of tension you have developed around the acts of sitting and standing (habits reflected in other everyday activities). Once aware of these patterns, you can begin consciously to direct your "use" of yourself as you sit and stand, and no longer rely on habits of muscular tension. Deceptively simple, these activities become more than a dynamic exercise for the support muscles of the back, they form your grounding in the skills of The Technique – skills that you can then apply to other, seemingly more complex, pursuits. Other explorations with your teacher will vary according to your particular interests.

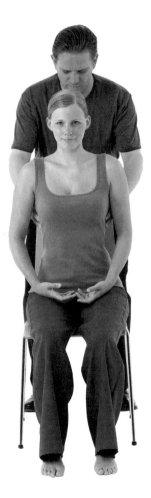

EXPLORING SITTING

An Alexander teacher guides you toward ways of sitting on a chair that will release ingrained habits of muscular tension. Try it now: sit on the front of a regular chair with your feet flat on the floor. Feel your sitting bones – the two bony parts of the pelvis beneath the flesh of your buttocks –against the seat. Let them support your weight. Keep your pelvis nicely upright, resisting the temptation to slump back, collapsing onto the back of your pelvis (this happens when the lower back is too weak to support the body). If you collapse in this way, place two similar-sized telephone directories beneath the back legs of the chair to angle the seat slightly, encouraging the pelvis to stay upright. Think of your weight falling through your sitting bones into the chair, like sand through an egg-timer. The more weight you allow to sink, the less you have to support through muscular effort. Consciously encourage your back muscles to release tension and open out, and think of your head moving up, away from the chair, while allowing your weight to drop down.

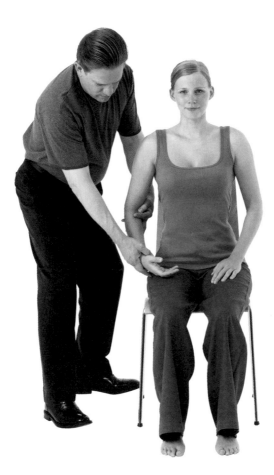

EXPLORING STANDING

Alexander teachers use touch and words to show you how to practise skills of The Technique while standing. Using your conscious mind in such an everyday action can be really effective in relieving frustration and discomfort.

Stand with your feet about hip-width apart, toes turned out slightly. Place one foot a little in front of the other (vary your foot position if you have to stand for long periods of time). Think about the floor rising beneath your feet, actively pushing you up as you allow both feet to spread out. Now think about the top of your head moving up, away from the soles of your feet. Thinking in this way creates stretch in the body's long muscles and makes space within the joints. Think of your weight dropping down through your entire body and finally through your feet into the earth below. When you stand on a moving surface, such as a bus or train, don't try to hold your weight away from the floor. This makes you top-heavy and less stable. Instead, ask your weight to move downward and don't resist the movement of the floor.

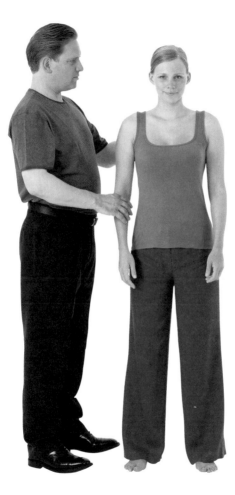

EXPLORING WALKING

Think about walking: does the way you move resemble weightless gliding, the pace and rhythm allowing you to think and be aware of your surroundings? Or does the movement feel clumsy, heavy or awkward? An Alexander teacher guides you as you learn how to walk truly upright in an effortless way. Experience it for yourself by taking a walk now and applying the following tips. First, don't stare at the ground. Instead, let your vision settle about 15m (50ft) ahead. Don't fix your gaze: let your eyes move naturally and "think" your head out in front of you. Now think about walking like an elephant: let your weight stay behind you as you move forward. Remain on your back foot, testing the ground before committing your weight to each step. This way of thinking can help to prevent stumbles. Experiment with thinking about objects coming toward you rather than you going to them, as if you are standing on a moving walkway. An Alexander teacher will offer further, personalized, ideas to help you to achieve easy, effortless forward motion.

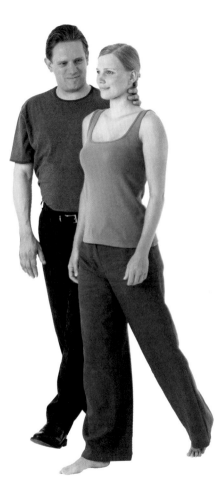

EXPLORING BENDING AND LIFTING

When bending to pick up an object, working at a surface or descending into a squat, many of us bend forward at the waist or upper back. The spine, however, does not have joints here, and so to do so can lead to slipped discs and permanent rounding of the upper back in older age. To maintain the integrity of the back, Alexander teachers help you to bend using your real joints: your ankles, knees and hips. Try it now with this practical exercise. Place an object about the size and weight of a soccer ball or shoe box on the floor. Stand close to the object, so that when your feet are shoulder-width apart it sits almost between your big toes. Bend at the knees and hips while directing your head, neck and back to lengthen so you fold up in a Z-shape. Bend low enough to grasp the soccer ball or box between your hands without stretching for it. Think of the object as connected to your back via your arms. Thinking in this way allows your whole body rather than the relatively weak arm muscles to absorb the load. Stand up, allowing the object to come up naturally with you.

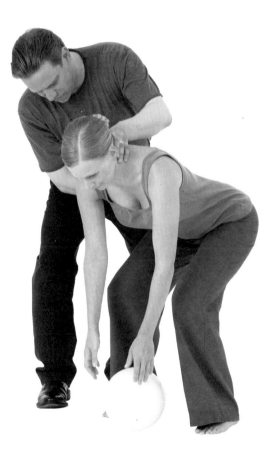

ENJOYING OTHER ACTIVITIES

Life is not about taking lessons. It's about movement: walking, talking, swimming, cycling, horseriding and countless other activities. Once you have acquired basic knowledge of The Alexander Technique, you can start to apply the skills to activities you love. Many Alexander teachers had a career in another field before training, and teach to reflect their own interests, so you might like to find one who shares your passions. My previous career was as an actor, so I frequently work with drama students and professional actors, combining my know-how and experience from both spheres. My lifelong love of bicycles has also led me to work with cyclists, both on and off the bike, helping them to get the most out of cycling. There are teachers working as musicians, swimming coaches and riding instructors, developing Alexander-based strategies for helping people to achieve their best playing an instrument, in the pool or on a horse. Many of these teachers run workshops or vacations catering for specific interests:

there are Alexander-orientated courses on everything from skiing to ballroom dancing. Residential breaks are an excellent way to explore subjects that interest you, and are more valuable when you have already gained experience of The Alexander Technique by taking lessons.

Within Alexander lessons you also explore all kinds of everyday activities – reading, writing, climbing stairs, doing housework or gardening – using perspectives gathered from learning the basics of The Technique. Rather than learning how to perform such daily actions "correctly", you find ways of acting without interfering in your overall "coherence". Then even the simplest act can benefit you rather than causing damage. Any well-trained Alexander teacher can teach you these skills; he or she does not have to share your interests. The specific activities you choose to explore together are simply a means to stimulate you and inhibit habitual reactions to stimuli – reactions that tend to involve making too much effort. Instead of learning how to do something right, you learn ways of acting and thinking that are simply more appropriate to various daily stimuli.

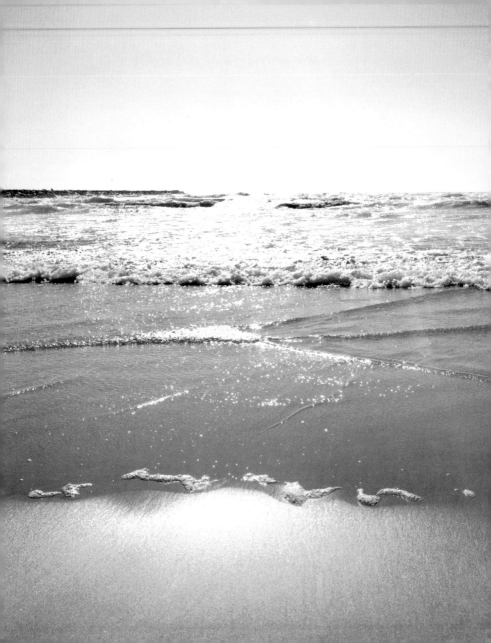

Change involves carrying out an activity
against the habit of life.

F.M. ALEXANDER

(1869–1955)

The universe is change;
our life is what our thoughts make it.

MARCUS AURELIUS

(121–180cc)

EXPLORING RELEASE

The Alexander Technique is about consciously guiding the way you use yourself in activity. But often those very activities have created the tensions you are working to undo, and between lessons old habits may try to take over. A useful means of continuing to change habits is to lie in a "semi-supine" position – flat on your back, with knees bent. Lying like this helps you to achieve a high level of muscular release throughout the body. Semi-supine work forms part of most Alexander lessons, lasting for a few minutes or much longer, according to the teacher, pupil and circumstances. You lie on a table (like a firm massage table) as the teacher gently uses his or her hands to achieve a muscular release that permits natural realignment. Most people find it deeply relaxing.

You can practise the exercise at home every day by following the steps on pages 118–119 – with tangible physical benefits. However, the benefits are greater if you work with a teacher, who combines lying down with effective Alexander "directions" (see pages 34–35).

Semi-supine exercise

1 Lie on your back on a firm surface – a folded blanket or exercise mat on a carpeted floor is ideal. Place your feet shoulder-width apart and close enough to your body that your knees point toward the ceiling. Rest your hands on your lower ribs or abdomen, elbows touching the floor.

2 Place a yoga block or pile of paperback books beneath your head for support. The height of the support is best determined by a teacher, but as a rough guide it should be high enough to angle your face slightly, so your chin is just lower than your forehead. Make contact with the support using the back of your skull, not your neck.

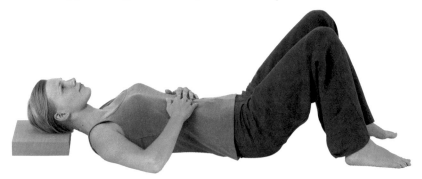

3 Become aware of your surroundings. What can you see and hear? Without cutting off this outside information, gently bring your attention to yourself. Become aware of sensations, such as heat and cold, tension and twitches. Allow these sensations to draw your awareness within.

4 While sustaining self-awareness, take your attention to your neck. Ask the muscles there to make less effort. Take your time; don't try to make anything happen.

5 Carry the instructions into the muscles running through your back. Allow yourself to be supported by the floor. Think of it lifting you as your back spreads in all directions. Allow the sense of opening to seep into your arms and legs so you expand from your centre. If your mind wanders, simply repeat the thought process.

6 Remain semi-supine for 15 to 20 minutes. To get up, roll onto all fours, allowing your spine to lengthen. Send your tail bone back to sit on your heels. "Think" your head up and let it lead you back onto your feet.

WHAT YOU TAKE AWAY
FROM A LESSON

Your experience of lessons in The Alexander Technique
will differ, to some extent, from anyone else's because
you are an individual. Yet students report many similar
reactions during and after sessions. My experiences as
a pupil were typical. I found early lessons mysterious.
The teacher didn't seem to do anything and yet I felt
bigger after a session – taller and wider – and lighter.
Walking down the street was akin to floating, as if someone were doing the action for me. There was a mailbox
on the corner of the street and, one day, after a lesson,
its colour seemed so bright I had to check it hadn't been
repainted. It was the same old box. I was also surprised
to experience discomfort in my back – not pain, more a
tired aching. I had never suffered from back problems.
I know now that this resulted from overworked muscles
undoing and other, under-exercised muscles waking up.
I was also often surprised at how "wrong" some actions
felt in lessons. I would feel as if I were leaning too far

backward, but, when the teacher turned me to look in the mirror, I was amazed to find myself standing perfectly upright. My habit was to lean forward, so being brought upright felt like falling backward, an effect of my faulty sensory appreciation (see pages 32–33).

I found the psychological changes most surprising. My confidence increased and I felt more able to express emotions freely and genuinely. My awareness was also enhanced. I recall lying on the table while my teacher worked on me, experiencing the notion of my whole back working as one piece. I had never "experienced" my back before. I used to work out at the gym, and so had large, overdeveloped muscles. These gradually became softer and smaller, yet stronger and better toned. Over the years, various health problems I had endured since childhood – asthma, hay fever and food sensitivities – gradually cleared up and my general health and vitality are now much improved. Your experiences of Alexander lessons will be different to mine (and, indeed, everyone else's), but I hope and expect they will be as remarkable, enjoyable and rewarding.

THE FUTURE OF THE TECHNIQUE

The Alexander Technique is about investing in the future by attending to the present. If you learn and apply the principles of The Technique now, you can prevent future problems (and resolve existing ones in the process). It follows that the earlier in life we learn to use ourselves well, the more chance there is of preventing problems that we associate with growing up and growing older.

Alexander believed the future of his work lay with children and education: it certainly has strong links with higher education through drama and music colleges. The Technique's future is also tied up with classification. It is often categorized as alternative therapy, but could more accurately be recognized as a system of education. Although it crosses many genres – health, psychology, movement, human potential, learning – in essence, The Technique is a unique way of taking responsibility for your future (not just limited to health issues). I urge you not to pigeonhole The Technique but, keeping an open mind, to experience it for yourself. You won't regret it.

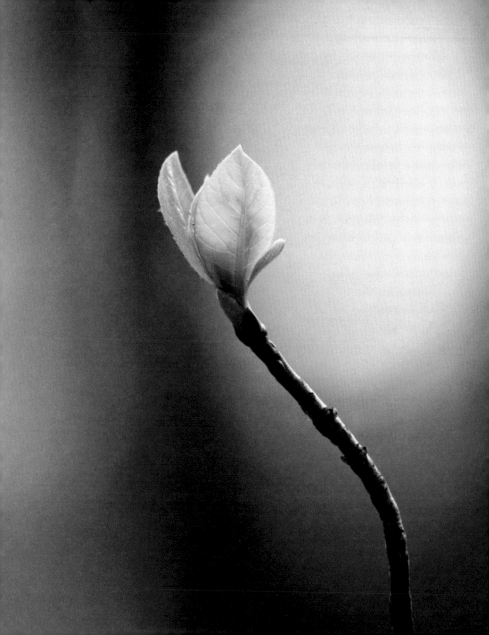

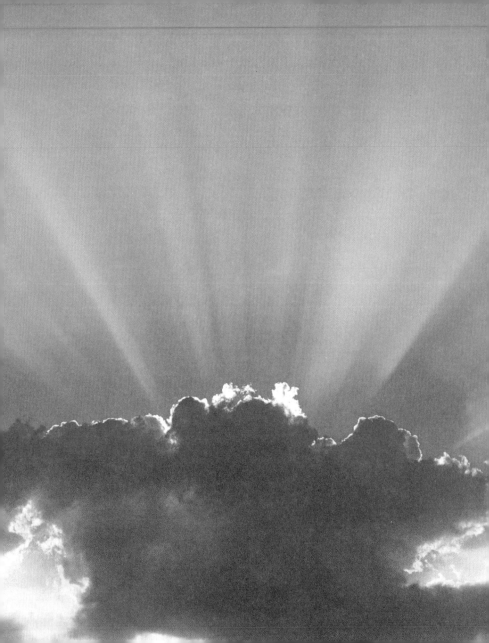

You must learn to be still in the midst of activity
and to be vibrantly alive in repose.

INDIRA GANDHI

(1917–84)

Compose yourself in stillness, draw your attention
inward and devote your mind to the Self.
The wisdom you seek lies within.

BHAGAVAD GITA

(c.50–500BCE)

INDEX

Picture Credits

The publisher would like to thank the following organizations and photographic libraries for permission to reproduce their material. Every care has been taken to trace copyright holders. However, if we have omitted anyone we apologize and will, if informed, make corrections to any future edition.

Page 2 Water Everywhere/Eyewire, **13** Earthforms/Digital Vision, **14** Photograph of F.M. Alexander © 2005, The Society of Teachers of the Alexander Technique, London, UK, **19** Ann Cutting/Botanica/ Photolibrary.com, **20** Natural Beauty EP018/Photodisc/Getty Images, **25** Hugh Sitton/Photographer's Choice/Getty Images, **26** Henry Steadman/Photolibrary.com, **29** Alexander Marius/Taxi/Getty Images, **37** Photos.com, **44** Zia Soleil/Iconica/Getty Images, **47** Peter Lewis/Alamy, **54** Natural Beauty EP018/ Photodisc/Getty Images, **57** John Freeman/Stone/Getty Images, **58** Frans Lemmens/Photographer's Choice/Getty Images, **61** David Paterson/Stone/Getty Images, **70** Angela Scott/Taxi/Getty Images, **73** John Gardey/Robert Harding World Imagery, London, **74** Hans Neleman/Photonica/Getty Images, **79** Stuart McClymont/Stone/Getty Images, **82** Mario Ponta/Alamy, **85** Jane Yeomans/Photonica/Getty Images, **86** Dana Edmunds/Pacific Stock/Photolibrary.com, **89** Natural Beauty EP018/Photodisc/Getty Images, **90** Art Wolfe/Imagebank/Getty Images, **114** Jacob Stock Photography/Photographer's Choice/ Getty Images, **117** John Churchman Veer/Photonica/Getty Images, **123** Ross M Horowitz/Iconica/Getty Images, **124** Peter Gridley/Taxi/Getty Images.

Text Credits

Quotations by F.M. Alexander, © The Estate of F.M. Alexander, courtesy of Mouritz Ltd, London.

Resources

For details of STAT-approved Alexander teachers working in the UK, search: www.stat.org.uk or phone 0845 230 7828.

To find STAT-approved teachers of The Alexander Technique in the US, search: www.alexandertech.org or phone 800 473 0620 or 413 584 2359.

To find STAT-affiliated societies around the world, go to: www.alexandertechniqueworldwide.com.

Author's Acknowledgments

To all my colleagues and students, with special thanks to Walter and Dilys Carrington and Suzi Morris.

Publisher's Acknowledgments

The publishers would like to thank: Model: Kate Mahoney Make-up artist: Gilly Popham